Galveston Diet For Seniors

Keys To Losing Weight And Regulating Your Hormonal Symptoms

By

Ella Anderson

TABLE OF CONTENT

INTRODUCTION

As we age, our bodies undergo many changes, including hormonal imbalances that contribute to weight gain and other health problems. The Galveston Diet for Seniors is a nutrition and lifestyle plan designed to help seniors lose weight, improve overall health, and manage hormonal symptoms. This diet is specially adapted to the special needs of the elderly. This e-book takes a closer look at the Galveston Diet and gives you the tools and knowledge you need to start your own health journey.

Chapter 1
Understanding Hormonal Imbalances In Seniors

As we age, our bodies undergo many changes, including hormonal imbalances that contribute to weight gain and other health problems. Hormonal changes in older adults can be caused by many factors, including menopause in women, menopause in men, and other medical conditions. Understanding these hormonal imbalances is essential to implementing an effective weight loss and health management plan like the Galveston Diet for Seniors. The Galveston Diet is specifically designed to help seniors manage hormonal imbalances and achieve their health and weight loss goals.

One of the major hormones that contribute to weight gain in older adults is estrogen. When a woman goes through menopause, her body produces less estrogen, which can lead to increased body fat and loss of muscle mass. The Galveston Diet emphasizes the importance of a balanced diet rich in protein to help maintain muscle mass and foods rich in phytoestrogens, such as soy products and flaxseed, to help control estrogen levels.

Another hormone that contributes to weight gain and other health problems in older adults is cortisol, produced by the adrenal glands in response to stress. Chronic stress can increase cortisol levels and cause fat to accumulate in the body, especially in the abdomen. The Galveston Diet advocates stress management techniques such as meditation and deep breathing, as well as regular exercise to help regulate cortisol levels. In addition to estrogen and cortisol, there are other hormones that contribute to weight gain and other health problems in older adults, such as insulin, thyroid hormones, and testosterone.

The Galveston Diet is designed to regulate these hormones through a balanced diet that includes nutritious whole foods and avoids processed and sugary foods.

Chapter 2
Galveston Diet Basics

The Galveston Diet for Seniors is a nutrition and lifestyle plan designed to help seniors lose weight, improve overall health, and manage hormonal symptoms. This diet, Dr. Mary Claire Haver is a board certified gynecologist and specially adapted to the special needs of seniors. The Galveston Diet is based on the principles of the Low Carb High Fat (LCHF) Diet, also known as the Ketogenic Diet, with some modifications.

The Galveston Diet emphasizes the importance of eating nutritious whole foods and avoiding processed and sugary foods. The diet is divided into three phases: an elimination phase, a transformation phase and a maintenance phase.

Deletion period
The elimination phase is the first phase of the Galveston diet and lasts 14 days. During this time, all processed foods, sugars and grains are removed from your diet. This period is designed to rehabilitate the body and help seniors break their addiction to sugar and processed foods. Older adults are encouraged to eat a variety of nutritious whole foods, including lean protein, healthy fats, and non-starchy vegetables. This period also encourages older adults to drink plenty of water and avoid alcohol and caffeine. conversion period

The Transformation Phase

It is the second phase of the Galveston Diet and lasts 10 weeks. In this stage, older people gradually reintroduce certain foods that were eliminated during the elimination stage, such as berries, nuts, and some grains. These steps are meant to help seniors find the right balance of carbohydrates, proteins, and fats to support weight loss and health goals. The Galveston Diet recommends that older adults eat one or two light meals three times a day, depending on how hungry they are. Older adults are encouraged to moderate their dietary intake and exercise regularly.

Maintenance period
The maintenance phase is the final phase of the Galveston Diet and is designed as a long-term lifestyle plan. During this time, older adults continue

to eat nutritious whole foods and maintain a balance of carbohydrates, proteins, and fats obtained during the transition period. Seniors are advised to continue to monitor their diet and exercise regularly to lose weight and maintain overall health. Beyond the three steps, the Galveston Diet emphasizes the importance of stress management and self-care. Seniors are encouraged to engage in stress-reducing activities, such as meditation, deep breathing or yoga, and to get enough sleep each night.

Chapter 3
Implementing The Galveston Diet

The Galveston Diet for Seniors requires some preparation and planning. Here are some tips to help seniors get started.

Talk to your healthcare provider
It is important to talk to your healthcare provider before starting any new diet or lifestyle plan, especially if you have any underlying medical conditions. Your doctor can determine if the Galveston diet is right for you and advise you on any necessary adjustments.

Eat nutritious whole foods

The Galveston Diet emphasizes the importance of eating nutritious whole foods, such as lean protein, healthy fats, and non-starchy vegetables. Older people should stock up on these types of foods and avoid processed and sugary foods.

plan a meal
Planning your meals ahead of time will help you stick to the Galveston Diet. Older adults should eat one or two light meals three times a day, depending on how hungry they are. Seniors can find recipe ideas and meal plans using resources like the Galveston Diet book or online resources.

Monitoring food intake
Tracking your food intake can help you stay accountable and meet the

recommended balance of carbohydrates, protein, and fat. Older adults can use resources such as food tracking apps or diaries to track their food intake.

Exercise regularly
Regular exercise is an important part of the Galveston diet. Older people should do at least 30 minutes a day of physical activity they enjoy, such as walking, swimming or yoga.

Practice stress management skills
Stress can have a negative impact on overall health and contribute to hormonal imbalance. Older adults should look to stress management techniques such as meditation, deep breathing, or yoga to reduce their stress levels. enough sleep

Getting enough sleep is important for overall health and helps regulate hormone levels. Seniors should aim for 7-9 hours of sleep per night.

Chapter 4
Overcoming Challenges And Staying On Track

Sticking to a new diet can be difficult, especially for older people who have to adjust to new dietary restrictions or habits. Here are some tips to help you overcome the challenges and stick to the Galveston Diet for Seniors.

Establishing specific objectives
When starting a new diet, it's important to set clear goals. Seniors should try small changes over time and focus on progress rather than perfection. Setting achievable goals can help older adults stay motivated and avoid excessive stress. planning social events

Social events can be difficult if you're trying to stick to a new diet. Seniors should plan ahead by bringing their own snacks or choosing healthy lunch options. They can also donate nutritional needs to friends and family to support social events.

Keep healthy snacks on hand
Having healthy snacks on hand can help seniors avoid temptation and stick to the Galveston Diet. Seniors can stock up on things like nuts, seeds and vegetables for quick and easy snacks.

Self-care practice
Practicing self-care can help older adults stay motivated and avoid emotional eating. Seniors can engage in activities such as yoga, meditation, or massage therapy to manage stress and improve overall well-being.

Use of support resources

The Galveston Diet Association offers a variety of resources and support to help seniors get on track. Seniors can connect with other dieters for motivation, support and recipe ideas.

Celebrate Progress

Celebrating accomplishments, no matter how small, can help seniors stay motivated and reach their goals. Seniors can reward themselves with non-food items, such as a new book or a relaxing bath, to recognize their accomplishments.

Seek professional help if necessary.

If older adults have problems following the Galveston diet or have problems with hormonal symptoms, they should seek professional help. A health care provider or dietitian can provide individualized guidance and support.

Chapter 5
Galveston Diet Success Stories

The Galveston Diet has helped many older adults achieve their health and weight loss goals. Here are some inspiring success stories from people who have followed the Galveston Diet.

Maria, 70

Mary struggled with weight gain and hormonal imbalance for several years. After hearing about the Galveston diet from a friend, she decided to give it a try. Within weeks, she noticed improvements in her energy levels, mood and hormonal symptoms. Within months, Mary lost 25 pounds and was able to maintain her weight loss by following the principles of the Galveston Diet.

Robert, 65 years old

Robert was diagnosed with type 2 diabetes and was trying to control his blood sugar. After starting the Galveston Diet, he saw significant improvements in his blood sugar levels and overall health. With the guidance of his healthcare provider, Robert was able to get off his diabetes medication and keep his blood sugar stable through a combination of diet and exercise.

Barbara, 72 years old

Barbara suffered from hot flashes and night sweats for years. After starting the Galveston Diet, she noticed a significant reduction in her symptoms. He also noticed improvements in sleep quality and general well-being. By following the Galveston Diet, Barbara was able to manage her hormonal symptoms without using hormone replacement therapy.

John ,68 years

John has suffered from high cholesterol and high blood pressure for many years. After starting the Galveston diet, she saw improvements in her cholesterol and blood pressure within weeks. Within months, John was able to reduce his medication and maintain healthy levels through a combination of diet and exercise.

 Sharon, 71 years old

Sharon has struggled with joint pain and inflammation for many years. After starting the Galveston diet, she experienced significant improvement in her joint pain and was able to reduce her use of anti-inflammatory medications. She also confirmed improvements in energy levels and overall quality of life.

CONCLUSION

The Galveston Diet for Seniors is a powerful tool to improve your health and quality of life as you age. Understanding your hormone imbalance, practicing the Galveston Diet, and overcoming challenges can help you achieve your weight loss and fitness goals. You can use the knowledge and resources provided in this e-book to take control of your health and begin your personal Galveston Diet journey.